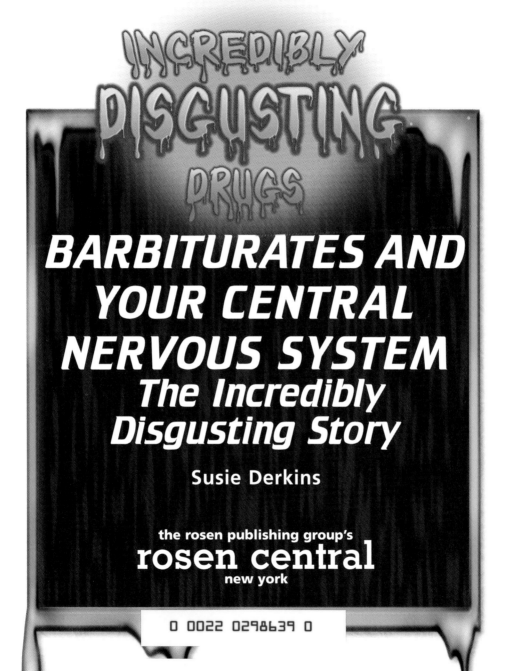

INCREDIBLY DISGUSTING DRUGS

BARBITURATES AND YOUR CENTRAL NERVOUS SYSTEM
The Incredibly Disgusting Story

Susie Derkins

the rosen publishing group's
rosen central
new york

Published in 2001 by The Rosen Publishing Group, Inc.
29 East 21st Street, New York, NY 10010

First Edition

Library of Congress Cataloging-in-Publication Data

Derkins, Susie.
Barbiturates and your central nervous system / by Susie Derkins.— 1st ed.
p. cm. — (Incredibly disgusting drugs)
Includes bibliographical references and index.
ISBN 0-8239-3388-1
1. Barbiturates—Juvenile literature. [1. Barbiturates. 2. Drug abuse.]
I. Title. II. Series.
RM325 .D47 2001
615'.782—dc21

2001000020

Manufactured in the United States of America

CONTENTS

Introduction

Do you know what barbiturates are? The use and abuse of barbiturates may not be as frequently discussed as heroin addiction, for example, or alcohol abuse. But barbiturates are indeed widely abused drugs, and barbiturates are extremely dangerous drugs—as potentially lethal as any other drug you can name.

Barbiturates are depressants, or downers, meaning that they dramatically slow down the body's functions (unlike stimulants, such as cocaine, which speed up bodily functions). Barbiturates, which usually come in brightly colored pills, tablets, or capsules, are available legally only with a doctor's prescription.

In high doses, barbiturates can be used for anesthesia—a state of extremely heavy sedation.

People undergoing surgery are anesthetized so that they will not feel any pain during an operation. However, in most cases, barbiturates are prescribed in much lower dosages to people who have problems such as insomnia, or trouble sleeping, or to people who are experiencing a short-term emotional crisis, such as a death in the family. This is because barbiturates can safely be taken only for very short periods of time.

The first problem with barbiturates is that users develop a tolerance for the drug very quickly, usually within two weeks. This means that the person will need to take more barbiturates, or a higher dosage of barbiturates, to achieve the original effects of the drug. And the more barbiturates a person takes, the higher the risk that he or she may ingest an amount that will cause an overdose.

The second problem with barbiturates is that they are extremely addictive. Addiction to barbiturates occurs just as quickly as tolerance develops. Once a person is addicted to barbiturates, he or she is in serious trouble. The difference between a dose of barbiturates that will lead to heavy sedation and one that will lead to coma or death is very, very slight. Many deaths have resulted from a barbiturate overdose, including those of incredibly

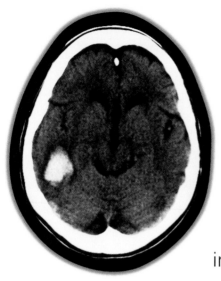

Using barbiturates can damage your brain.

talented people such as film icon Marilyn Monroe, rock legend Jimi Hendrix, and comedian Chris Farley.

If other depressant drugs, such as alcohol or heroin, are taken with barbiturates the risk of overdose increases dramatically. It is even dangerous for a person to try to stop using barbiturates because of the specific effects that the drug has on the body's central nervous system—the system that controls brain and spine functions, among other things. Withdrawing from using barbiturates is so risky that it can be done safely only under close medical supervision.

This book will explain the dangers of barbiturate use and abuse. First, we will talk about what barbiturates are, including how they are classified and how they affect the body at different dosages. We will look at some of the reasons why people start to use barbiturates and how this use can easily lead to abuse. We will also discuss some drugs that have been developed as alternatives to barbiturates but that can also be problematic when abused.

Later on, we will explain how barbiturates affect the body's central nervous system (CNS) functions, most specifically those of the brain. The last chapter of this book will describe the process of overdose and the stages and dangers of barbiturate withdrawal. There is also a Where to Go for Help section at the back of this book that provides resource information, in case you or someone you know needs further information or help.

The use of barbiturates is as potentially hazardous as the use of heroin, crack, alcohol, or any other drug. The havoc that barbiturates can create in the body's central nervous system needs to be understood because even a small dosage of barbiturates can cause coma or a fatal overdose.

1 What Are Barbiturates?

Most drugs—including those that are highly addictive, dangerous, and frequently abused—were first used or developed for medicinal and scientific purposes. This includes the family of drugs known as barbiturates.

Adolf von Baeyer, a German pharmacist of the nineteenth century, oversaw a laboratory where many important cures and treatments for disease and pain were discovered or developed. For example, Baeyer's pharmaceutical firm pioneered the use of opiates for the treatment of pain. Baeyer's lab was also where aspirin was developed. To this day, Bayer Aspirin can be found on drugstore shelves around the world.

In 1862, Baeyer's lab combined urea (a solution made from animal urine) and malonic acid

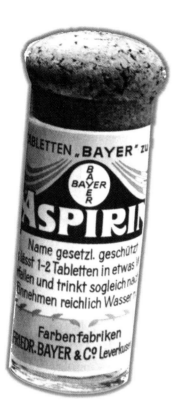

The maker of Bayer developed opiates for the treatment of pain.

(a type of acid that comes from fruit) to make barbituric acid. The compound was dubbed "Barbara's urates" after Saint Barbara, the patron saint of December 4, the day the compound was made.

At first, the makers of Bayer were unsure of how to best utilize their new drug compound. But by 1903, Barbara's urates were being used by doctors for sedation, or to induce sleep. They were also used for anesthesia during surgery. (Anesthesia drugs heavily sedate the body, so a patient will not feel any pain during surgery.) Soon, barbiturates were being prescribed for many different ailments, such as nervousness and insomnia.

Phenobarbital, a popular type of barbiturate, was widely available by prescription by 1912.

Barbiturates helped to sedate the fidgety and reduce the frequency of seizures in epileptics. The drugs were regularly used to calm traumatized patients in mental hospitals, to anesthetize people for operations, and to treat people who suffered from convulsions. More than 2,500 different types of barbiturates have been developed from Baeyer's original formula.

However, barbiturates are clearly not the wonder drug they seemed almost a century ago. Most important, barbiturates were quickly found to be highly addictive. When a person begins to take barbiturates on a regular basis, he or she will develop a tolerance for them. Tolerance develops when a person repeatedly uses a drug; over time, his or her body becomes less responsive to the drug's effects. This means that the user must take increasing amounts of the drug to produce the desired effects.

Developing a tolerance to any drug is risky, but when it comes to barbiturates, the tolerance that results from regular use is extremely dangerous. Regular abuse of barbiturates can cause a complete breakdown of the body's central nervous system (CNS)—the system that is responsible for the proper function of your brain and

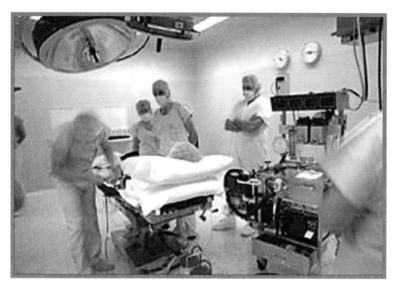
Barbiturates have been used for surgery to anesthetize people so they don't feel any pain.

spinal cord. Damage to the central nervous system can result in coma and even death.

There is only a tiny difference between a dose of barbiturates that will lead to heavy sedation and one that will lead to an overdose or coma. This is even more true when other depressant drugs, such as alcohol or heroin, are added to the mix. Many deaths have resulted when a barbiturate user falls into the tiny sliver of unconsciousness right before a fatal overdose. Once a person has fallen into that state, he or she will quickly experience respiratory failure—which means that the lungs can no longer function properly and the person stops breathing.

Sometimes, because a high dosage of barbiturates has left the user unconscious and unable to move, he or she will suffocate by choking to death on vomit.

Once a person is addicted to barbiturates, he or she risks death on a daily basis, but users also risk death during attempts to withdraw from the drug. Withdrawal, or the process of discontinuing the use of a drug to which he or she is addicted, is a dangerous process for a barbiturate addict. There is a very high risk of seizure, coma, and death during the grueling process of barbiturate withdrawal.

IF BARBITURATES ARE SO DANGEROUS . . .

If barbiturates are so dangerous, why do doctors continue to prescribe them? Doctors prescribe depressant drugs to people who experience insomnia and anxiety. Most depressant drugs prescribed today are not barbiturates, however, but are other drugs called benzodiazepines, or minor tranquilizers. Benzodiazepines, such as Rohypnol and Valium, are considered less addictive and less potent, or strong, than barbiturates. (We'll talk about the specific differences between these drugs and barbiturates in chapter 2.)

Benzodiazepines were developed as alternative central nervous system depressants because barbiturates were widely considered to be too risky. Only about 20 percent of depressant prescriptions written today are for barbiturates. However, barbiturates are still regularly used to treat some kinds of epilepsy. And they are widely manufactured, sold, and abused illegally. Barbiturates have always played a major part in suicides and accidental overdoses. And they have a considerably higher potential for addiction than do benzodiazepines.

BARBITURATE CLASSIFICATION

Barbiturates are sometimes called hypnosedatives. This term comes from the names of two drug classifications: hypnotics, which act as sleeping pills, and sedatives, which are used to calm people down. While there are currently more than 2,000 known barbiturates sold under hundreds of trade names, they are all based upon the same basic chemical recipe. Fewer than twenty variations of Adolf von Baeyer's original compound are commonly used today.

In similar dosages, different barbiturates have basically similar effects on the body. Barbiturates are usually classified into one of three different groups, depending on how fast they begin to work and how long the effects last.

Ultrashort-acting barbiturates produce quick effects, usually within twenty minutes. They are typically used to prepare surgery patients by calming them before administering full anesthesia. Effects last from three to six hours.

Short-acting or intermediate-acting barbiturates take slightly longer to achieve their effects, but they also work for a longer period of time—about six to ten hours. These drugs are often prescribed to people who have trouble sleeping, and they are also the group of barbiturates most subject to abuse.

Long-acting barbiturates may not take effect in the body for hours or even days. They are usually prescribed for people who suffer from epileptic seizures.

DOSAGES

Barbiturates can be further categorized by the strength of a particular prescription's dosage. Behavioral effects of barbiturates are different, depending on the amount of the drug in the body. Low dosages are 50 milligrams or less. The effect of this amount of barbiturates is similar to alcohol intoxication. Memory, coordination, and speech are slightly impaired. Anxiety is reduced. Respiration, or the rate at which you breathe, slows down as your blood pressure and your heart rate drop.

COMMON BARBITURATE NAMES

● Trade names: Amytal, Butisol, Nembutal, Seconal, Tuinal.

● Generic names: amobarbital, butabarbital, pentobarbital ("truth serum"), phenobarbital, secobarbital.

● Street names: barbs, downers, sleepers, blues, yellow jackets, red devils, purple hearts.

● Note: Quaaludes ("ludes") are NOT barbiturates. They are called nonbarbiturate sedative-hypnotics and were designed to be safe alternatives to the old barbiturates. However, most nonbarbiturate sedative-hypnotics are as addictive and nearly as dangerous as the barbiturates they were designed to replace.

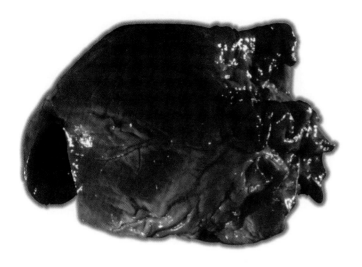

High doses of barbiturates can cause a user's heart to stop working.

Moderate dosages are 100 to 200 milligrams. The sedative effects of barbiturates are more obvious at this dosage. Users tend to sleep deeply and frequently. Slurred speech and impaired judgment may also result. (For more information about the effect of barbiturates on the brain and the body's functions, see chapter 3.)

High dosages are 200 milligrams or more. In a non-addicted person, a high dosage of barbiturates can cause very dramatic and unpredictable levels of intoxication. Common effects include intense mood swings, babbling or incoherent speech, and a lack of coordination and judgment. Blood pressure can drop so dangerously low that a person has a cardiovascular collapse. In an already addicted person, high dosages and even medium dosages can easily lead to excessive sedation and even coma and death.

2 Why Do People Use Barbiturates?

Barbiturates are depressants, and depressants act as "downers." Depressant drugs, such as barbiturates or alcohol, slow down the body's functions (unlike stimulant drugs, such as cocaine or caffeine, which speed up bodily functions). Barbiturates are available legally only with a doctor's prescription. They usually come in pills, tablets, or capsules, and are often brightly colored.

At first, a small dose of barbiturates will help an insomniac to sleep. But that dosage typically loses its effectiveness very quickly—the original effects start to wear off in about two weeks. Unless a person stops using the drug, he or she will have to up the dosage of barbiturates to achieve the drug's original effect. At

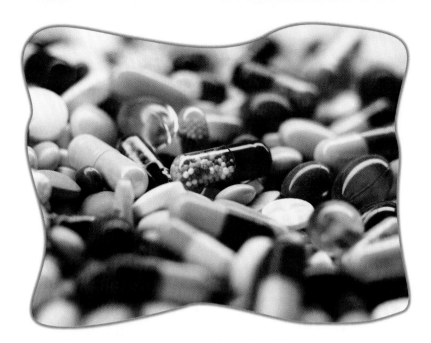

Barbiturates are prescribed for legitimate
medical reasons, but users can become abusers.

this stage, it can be said that the person has developed
a physical tolerance to the drug. Once that physical
tolerance has developed, the sliver of time between deep
sleep and a fatal overdose becomes extremely narrow.

Barbiturates, if not prescribed for seizures or anesthesia,
are meant to be taken only for a very limited period of
time. Doctors may prescribe them to patients who are
coping with a particular crisis, such as a sudden death in
the family. But sometimes a person will take his or her
pills more frequently than is recommended by a doctor, or
take more pills at one time than the doctor prescribes.

Eventually, the person may lie to his or her doctor and say that it is still difficult to sleep, or that the dosage is wearing off and needs to be increased. This is because the user is hoping to get more pills or a stronger prescription.

WHY DO PEOPLE ABUSE BARBITURATES?

Some people simply use barbiturates for a high. They buy them off the street or steal them from someone who has a legal prescription. Some addicts and dealers have even broken into drugstores looking for barbiturates to take or sell on the street. Other people steal doctors' prescription pads and attempt to write out false prescriptions. Robbing drugstores and forging prescriptions are serious crimes. But some addicts will do these things anyway because the impulse to get more barbiturates is so strong and because barbiturate addiction is that severe.

At first, barbiturates may make one feel peaceful, extremely relaxed, and free from physical pain. But after barbiturates have been used over a period of time, a user's behavior becomes erratic. He or she will experience a regular loss of memory and judgment, as well as mood swings, depression, and extreme fatigue. A user almost always loses the desire to care for himself or herself. Soon enough, family members, friends, jobs, and appearance are neglected. It is not uncommon for barbiturate abusers to become paranoid or to develop suicidal thoughts.

INJECTING BARBITURATES

Some barbiturate abusers prepare the powder inside barbiturate pills for injection. They cook the powder with water to form a liquid—and deadly—form of the drug. Once injected into a vein, the effect of the drug is instant, causing full-body warmth and extreme drowsiness.

While barbiturates are most commonly taken in the form of pills or tablets, many people who are long-term, high-dosage barbiturate abusers eventually begin injecting the drug. When a drug is injected directly into the bloodstream, its effect is almost immediate and is much stronger and more intense than if it is taken by mouth—at least until a tolerance has been developed.

Injection of any drug is extremely dangerous, and overdose is an all-too-common result. Gangrene, or death of the body's skin tissue, and abscesses, or disease-plagued lesions, often occur at the spot where the drug is injected. In addition, drug users who share needles with other users put themselves at serious risk of contracting diseases such as hepatitis. Sharing needles is also a high-risk behavior because it is a primary way to spread the human immunodeficiency virus (HIV), the virus that causes AIDS.

BENZODIAZEPINES, OR MINOR TRANQUILIZERS

Benzodiazepines, sometimes called minor tranquilizers, were created as a less risky replacement for barbiturates. Developed in the 1960s, they were created so users would have less risk of addiction and overdose. Common brands of benzodiazepines include Valium, Xanax, and Librium. While benzodiazepines are generally safe, many people abuse these drugs just as barbiturates are abused, and it is entirely

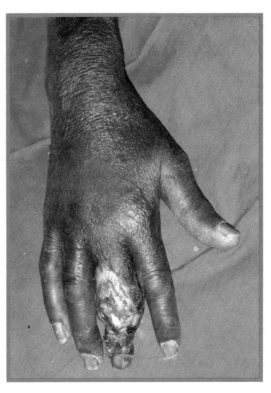

Injecting barbiturates can cause gangrene, which rots tissues.

BARBITURATE DEATH: MARILYN MONROE

The legendary film icon Marilyn Monroe was found dead of a barbiturate overdose in 1962. The official report of her death was suicide by sleeping pills, although controversy surrounds the cause of her death. Many people believe that the overdose was accidental or possibly even administered by someone other than Monroe for political reasons. (She had been romantically linked to two prominent politicians, President John F. Kennedy and his brother Attorney General Robert Kennedy.)

Voted the top star of 1952 by American film distributors, Marilyn rocketed to fame in films like Bus Stop, Some Like It Hot, and The Misfits. To this day, she is beloved by millions worldwide for her timeless, exceptional beauty, and the films and footage that showcase her charm and comedic gifts.

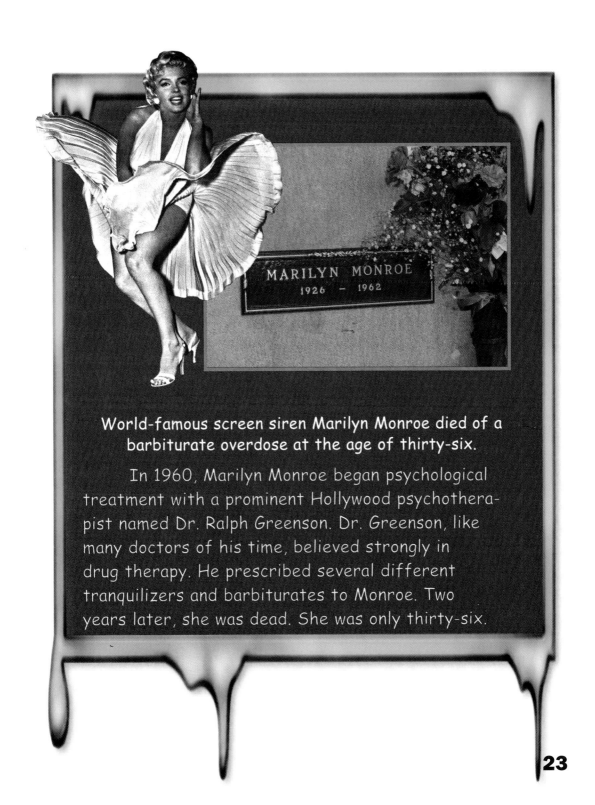

World-famous screen siren Marilyn Monroe died of a barbiturate overdose at the age of thirty-six.

In 1960, Marilyn Monroe began psychological treatment with a prominent Hollywood psychotherapist named Dr. Ralph Greenson. Dr. Greenson, like many doctors of his time, believed strongly in drug therapy. He prescribed several different tranquilizers and barbiturates to Monroe. Two years later, she was dead. She was only thirty-six.

possible to become both psychologically and physically addicted to them as well. Much like barbiturates, benzodiazepines are especially dangerous when combined with other drugs, particularly other CNS depressants such as alcohol or heroin.

Benzodiazepines may not be as strong or as potentially dangerous as many of the barbiturates they replaced, but they are hardly safe. Valium, for instance, has a very long history of abuse. The abuse of, and addiction to, these "minor" tranquilizers has been dramatically depicted in films such as *Drugstore Cowboy* and *Valley of the Dolls*. Benzodiazepines are very commonly prescribed drugs, and they continue to be one of the drugs most frequently connected with emergency-room visits caused by drug overdose.

Clearly, unless you are under close medical supervision, it is best to just stay away from depressants—alcohol, tranquilizers, and especially barbiturates.

A HISTORY OF ABUSE

Barbiturates and benzodiazepines also have a history of having been heavily prescribed to women. Beginning in the 1950s, doctors began to write out a large number of

prescriptions for barbiturates and benzodiazepines,
particularly to middle-class
American women. Instead
of being prescribed simply
to help a woman deal
with a short-term crisis or
a period of extreme
depression or anxiety,
these drugs were given to
women to treat "prob-
lems" such as daily stress,
boredom, loneliness, and
family difficulties.
However, the danger-
ously high tolerance
and addiction rates of

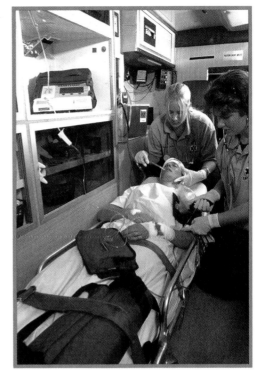

Sometimes, abusing
benzodiazepines results in
drug overdoses.

these drugs make them unsuitable for daily use, and
many women became addicted to the drugs as a result.
Even today, women are a high-risk group for tranquilizer
and barbiturate abuse. According to the National
Institute on Drug Abuse, 3.7 million women took prescription drugs for nonmedical reasons last year.

3 Barbiturates and Your Central Nervous System

The body's central nervous system is composed of the brain and spinal cord. Sensory impulses that control motor skills, such as speech and coordination, are transmitted through this complex network.

Barbiturates depress the brain's functions. Short-term barbiturate abuse causes impaired thinking, memory, and judgment. Barbiturates also mess with a person's reflexes, so that physical reactions are not as quick, and they cause chronic and severe fatigue. Barbiturates slow down the body's central nervous system, depressing normal body and brain functioning. As soon as barbiturates enter the bloodstream, they lower the body's blood pressure, heart rate, and respiratory rate.

It gets even worse. Short-term barbiturate abuse almost always leads to long-term abuse because the drugs are so powerfully addictive. Barbiturate abusers often find themselves feeling depressed, hostile, paranoid, disoriented, and suicidal. Over time, their central nervous systems deteriorate, permanently damaged by toxic levels of barbiturates. And it is far from uncommon to see barbiturate abuse result in death from accidental overdose.

THE CENTRAL NERVOUS SYSTEM (CNS)

The central nervous system can be divided into two major parts: the brain and the spinal cord. The brain contains more than 100 billion nerve cells, called neurons, that are responsible for sending information to different parts of the brain. Damage to the brain's major parts—the cerebellum and the cerebral cortex—can result in a loss of all kinds of basic bodily functions. This is because the cerebral cortex is responsible for thought, voluntary movements, speech, reasoning, and perception. The cerebellum controls the body's movement, balance, and posture.

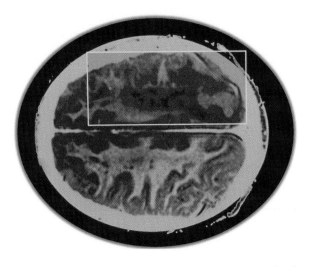

Brain damage can devastate many of the body's basic functions, such as speech.

The brain connects to the spine at a point known as the brain stem. The brain stem connects the brain to the thalamus. The thalamus is the body's little information center: It receives sensory information from the cerebral cortex and transmits this information through neurons to other parts of the brain and spine. It also fires neurons back to the cerebral cortex. The thalamus is responsible for proper functioning of the senses and for basic motor skills, such as eye-hand coordination and speech. A smaller section of the thalamus, called the hypothalamus, regulates body temperature, emotions, hunger, and thirst. All of these organs and basic bodily functions are put at risk when barbiturates cross the brain's protective layer.

BLOOD BRAIN BARRIER (BBB)

The brain has what is called a blood brain barrier, or BBB. The BBB is a lipid (fatty) layer that surrounds the brain, preventing foreign substances in the bloodstream from entering the brain and causing malfunctions. The BBB is semi-permeable, meaning that some materials can cross the barrier, while others cannot. In this way, the BBB helps the brain to maintain a constant, or regular, environment. Large

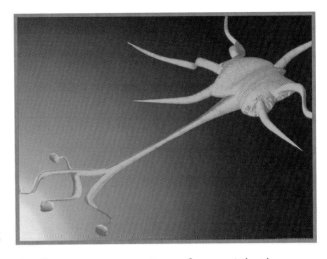

Barbiturates may interfere with the flow of data across the brain's neurons.

molecules do not pass easily through the BBB, nor do molecules that cannot dissolve easily in fat.

Depressant drugs, such as alcohol and barbiturates, dissolve easily in fat, giving them access to the brain when the BBB is permeated, or crossed. Drugs that are dissolved easily in fat can also accumulate in the body's fatty tissue and reenter the bloodstream later. Different barbiturates may clear out of the bloodstream at different rates, depending upon their potency. Researchers believe that barbiturates bind to sodium channels on neurons—the cells that tell the brain what data to transmit—and prevent the flow of sodium ions. When sodium ions cannot flow across the neuronal membrane, the brain cannot tell the body how to function.

THE EFFECTS OF BARBITURATES ON THE BODY

Let's take a closer look at how barbiturates physically affect the body after they penetrate the blood brain barrier and enter the bloodstream.

LOSS OF INHIBITIONS

The first reaction after a person has ingested barbiturates is a lessening of inhibitions. Inhibitions are emotions or instincts that tell you to restrict your behavior or restrain your expressions. It can sometimes feel good to lose your inhibitions because feeling uninhibited means feeling relaxed. Although a loosening of inhibitions is not as dangerous as the effects felt when taking depressant drugs at higher dosages, it is still risky behavior. This is because inhibitions are the body's way of controlling itself, both physically and psychologically. A loss of inhibitions can cause you to act in ways that you normally wouldn't. You may find yourself taking dangerous risks, or worse, ignoring signals that you have already ingested a toxic level of a drug. And after you have taken a lot of barbiturates and are no longer able to tell exactly how messed up you have become, you are inviting an overdose.

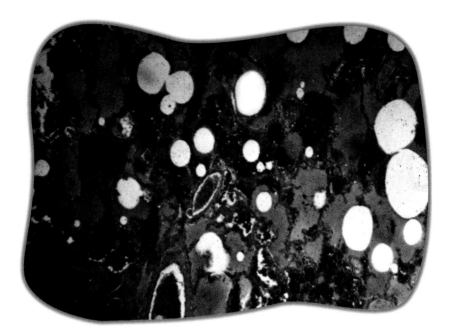

After barbiturates cross the blood brain barrier, they can wreak havoc on the user's mind and body.

HEAVY SEDATION

After the initial high, the barbiturate user begins to feel very fatigued and drowsy. Users slur their speech and experience slowed responses or actions. Their eyes become unfocused, and they may stagger or move unsteadily. This is a very unsafe stage in the barbiturate high, especially if barbiturates are not the only depressant that a person has ingested. Sometimes, the body will try to reject an excessive amount of pills or alcohol through vomiting. But if a barbiturate user is lying on his or her back, and is too sedated to get up, he or she may choke to death, suffocating on vomit.

BARBITURATE DEATH: JIMI HENDRIX

Pioneering guitarist and rock legend Jimi Hendrix died in 1970 at the age of twenty-seven from a barbiturate overdose. Born Johnny Allen Hendrix in Seattle, Washington, Jimi Hendrix has been more highly praised than any other rock guitarist and remains a tremendous influence on musicians to this day. Hendrix is probably best known for the album Are You Experienced? He was also a major star of the original Woodstock Festival in 1969, where he made history with an electrified version of the "Star-Spangled Banner."

Earlier in the day that Jimi Hendrix died, his girlfriend had become alarmed when she was unable to rouse him from a deep sleep. An ambulance was called, but Hendrix was pronounced dead on arrival at a nearby

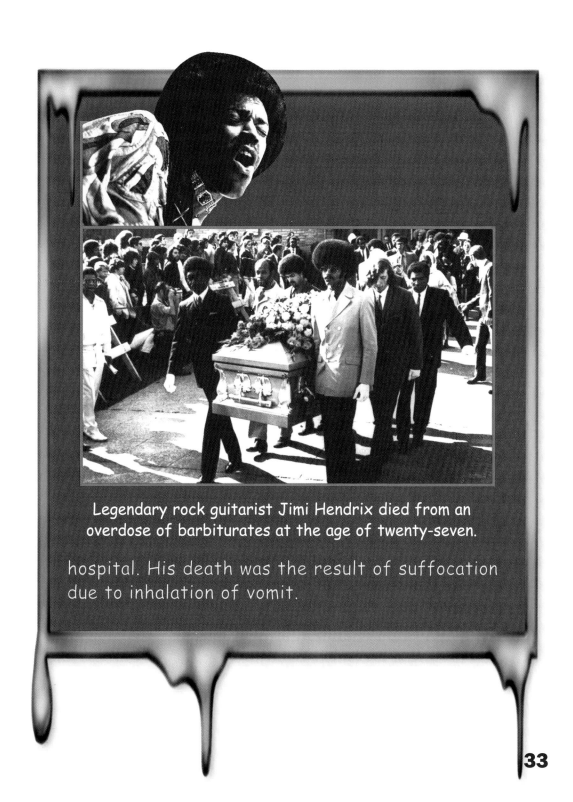

Legendary rock guitarist Jimi Hendrix died from an overdose of barbiturates at the age of twenty-seven.

hospital. His death was the result of suffocation due to inhalation of vomit.

RESPIRATORY ARREST AND COMA

A barbiturate overdose can slow the heart and respiratory rates so dramatically that a person will simply stop breathing. Blood fails to flow quickly enough to the heart and the brain, and the central nervous system shuts down. At this point, the user will fall into a coma, a state of profound unconsciousness. A similar reaction is common when barbiturates are taken with other central nervous system depressants, such as alcohol, heroin, morphine, or codeine. Even antihistamine drugs, such as over-the-counter allergy and cold medications, are extremely dangerous when taken with barbiturates because they also depress the central nervous system and can lead to respiratory arrest.

It cannot be stated too many times: Barbiturates are extremely dangerous on their own, but when mixed with other drugs, they can cause deadly results in a very short period of time. A combination of drugs, such as alcohol and barbiturates, is a lethal cocktail, a recipe for death. More than half of all accidental overdoses result from mixing depressant drugs with alcohol. Perhaps this is because users do not realize the extremely dangerous "pile-up," or multiplying effect, that depressants can have when taken together. Alcohol intensifies any existing intoxication and is especially lethal when mixed with barbiturates.

barbiturates is not easy, but it's much less painful than continuing down the road of addiction. The longer one has been using barbiturates, the worse the effects of withdrawal, so users are advised to quit as soon as possible.

In the hospital, the patient will be evaluated physically and mentally; he or she will be given a drug test to see what substances are in his or her system. Once it has been determined which drugs are present in the system, detoxification can begin. This can be accomplished by giving the patient lower and lower doses of the drug, slowly and gently weaning the person off the substance. Or a doctor may use a substitute drug that has effects similar to the barbiturate but with less severe withdrawal symptoms. This can be done only under the careful and controlled supervision of doctors and medical professionals. Otherwise, it is entirely possible for an addict to become addicted to the drug that was supposed to help him or her beat the initial addiction.

Barbiturate withdrawal symptoms usually kick in within seventy-two hours of the last dose, but this varies somewhat depending on how large the last dose was, a person's tolerance to the particular drug and potency, and the person's physical condition and size. The first stage of barbiturate withdrawal includes insomnia,

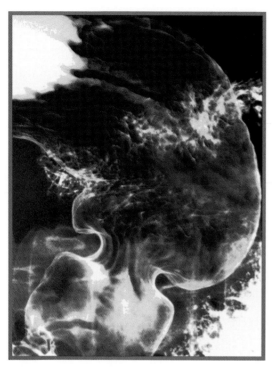

Withdrawing from barbiturates will affect your entire body.

anxiety, and low-grade fever. The second stage involves more of those same symptoms, plus hallucinations, vomiting, and uncontrollable shaking. The third stage includes a high-grade fever and extreme disori-entation—not having any idea of where one is, for example. At this stage, the user may not recognize family members, friends, or other loved ones. The person may not understand anything about what is hap-pening to him or her.

It is important to remember that barbiturate-overdose deaths can occur at any of these three stages. In fact, many users have experienced coma and death during the first stage of withdrawal. That is why it is crucial that a person not try to withdraw from barbiturates on his or her own. It is always recommended that a person be in the hospital before any symptoms of withdrawal begin.

BARBITURATE DEATH: CHRIS FARLEY

Chris Farley, the outrageous stand-up comedian and actor best known for his work on Saturday Night Live, died in a Chicago hotel room on December 18, 1998, of a heart attack brought on by a combination of barbiturates and alcohol. He was thirty-three.

Chris Farley's unique style of physical comedy won him many fans. After joining Saturday Night Live in 1990, Farley appeared in movies such as Wayne's World and Coneheads, as well as Tommy Boy and Black Sheep with his friend David Spade.

Farley was born and raised in Madison, Wisconsin. He attended Marquette University, earning a degree in communications and theater. He performed with local improv groups until he was discovered at Chicago's Second City Theater by SNL producer Lorne Michaels. Ironically, Chris Farley's hero, SNL legend John Belushi, also died at the age of thirty-three of a heart attack that was drug-induced.

Even if withdrawal doesn't kill a person, he or she may wish that it would. Withdrawal from barbiturates is horrible, frightening, and lengthy—usually about seventy-two hours, or three days. Additional symptoms include mental anguish (including frightening hallucinations), chills, severe cramps, convulsions, nausea, vomiting, insomnia, and delirium.

GETTING HELP

After the withdrawal and detoxification process, barbiturate users will still need a lot of help. The psychological aspects of addiction, such as long-term depression or fear, must be addressed. Major life changes, such as breaking away from old friends or circumstances, are almost always required. Therapy and strong group support are especially effective in helping users avoid a relapse, which is common when someone is trying to stay off any type of drug.

If you or someone you know needs help with an addiction to barbiturates, seek help. Talk to a parent or another trusted adult, such as a teacher, school counselor, or psychologist. There are also helpful Web sites and hotlines listed in the Where to Go for Help section at the back of this book. Help is out there. Don't be afraid to ask for it. Your life, or the life of someone you love, may depend on it.

GLOSSARY

abscesses Infected lesions on the skin, often found at the point where a drug user has repeatedly injected a drug into his or her body.

addiction A compulsive physical and/or psychological need for and use of a habit-forming substance, such as alcohol or tranquilizers.

anesthesia A state of extremely heavy sedation. Surgery patients are regularly anesthetized so that they will not feel any pain or discomfort as an operation is being performed.

barbiturate A depressant and highly addicting drug used as a sedative or anesthetic.

brain stem The part of the brain that connects the spinal cord to the cerebellum.

central nervous system (CNS) The system of the body, including the brain and spinal cord, through which sensory impulses are transmitted to control motor skills.

coma A state of profound unconsciousness that can be brought about by an overdose of barbiturates.

depressant drugs Drugs, such as barbiturates or alcohol, that reduce or slow down bodily functions and activity.

detoxification The process of freeing a drug user from a physical substance addiction.

gangrene   Complete death of skin tissue because of lack of blood flow.

inhibitions   Emotions or inner instincts that tell you to restrict your actions or restrain your behavior.

insomnia   Inability to sleep.

neurons   Special brain cells that tell the brain what information to transmit throughout the central nervous system.

overdose   A lethal, or deadly, amount of a drug that can lead to coma or death.

relapse   The act of using or abusing drugs after a period of improvement or abstinence.

sedation   The state of extreme calm or fatigue that results from the use of sedative drugs, such as sleeping pills.

stimulant drugs   Drugs, such as cocaine or caffeine, that increase or speed up bodily functions and activity.

thalamus   Part of the brain responsible for the processing of sensory information.

tolerance   When the body becomes less responsive to a drug's effects because of repeated use of the drug.

unconscious   A state of not having conscious thought or awareness; being "passed out."

withdrawal   A method of discontinuing the use of a drug or other addictive substance.

FOR MORE INFORMATION

In the United States

Food and Drug Administration
    (FDA)
5600 Fishers Lane
Rockville, MD 20857
(888) INFO-FDA (463-6332)
e-mail: webmail@fda.gov
Web site: http://www.fda.gov

Partnership for a
    Drug-Free America
405 Lexington Avenue
16th Floor
(212) 922-1560
New York, NY 10174
Web site:
    http://drugfreeamerica.org

In Canada

Canadian Centre on
    Substance Abuse
75 Albert Street, Suite 300
Ottawa, ON K1P 5E7
(613) 235-4048
Web site: http://www.ccsa.ca

Toronto Area Committee of
    Narcotics Anonymous
Box 5700, Depot A
Toronto, ON M5W 1N8
(416) 236-8956
Web site: http://www.
    members.better.net/
    toronto_na

Web Sites

Due to the changing nature of
Internet links, the Rosen
Publishing Group, Inc., has
developed an online list of
Web sites related to the
subject of this book. This site
is updated regularly. Please
use this link to access the list:

http://www.rosenlinks.com/
    idd/bcns

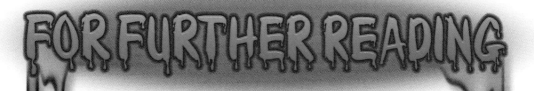

FOR FURTHER READING

Anonymous. *Go Ask Alice*. New York: Aladdin Paperbacks, 1998.

Clayton, Lawrence. *Barbiturates and Other Depressants*. Rev. ed. New York: The Rosen Publishing Group, Inc.,1998.

Gordon, Melanie Apel. *Drug Interactions: Protecting Yourself from Dangerous Drug, Medication, and Food Combinations*. New York: The Rosen Publishing Group, Inc.,1999.

Graedon, Joe, and Teresa Graedon. *The People's Guide to Deadly Drug Interactions*. New York: St. Martin's Press, 1995.

Mass, Wendy. *Teen Drug Abuse*. San Diego, CA: Lucent Books, 1998.

McLaughlin, Miriam Smith. *Addiction: The "High" That Brings You Down*. Springfield, NJ: Enslow Publishers, 1997.

Roberts, Jeremy. *Prescription Drug Abuse*. New York: The Rosen Publishing Group, Inc., 2000.

INDEX

CREDITS

About the Author

Susie Derkins is a writer and artist who lives in New York City's East Village. She is currently working on a novel.

Photo Credits

Cover © SuperStock; p. 6 © Scott Camazine/Photo Researchers, Inc.; p. 9 © Associated Press; p. 11 © Terry Oakley/The Picture Source; p. 16 © Photo Researchers, Inc.; p. 18 © SuperStock; p. 21 © CMSP; p. 23 © Associated Press; p. 25 © Bill Bachmann/Index Stock; pp. 28, 29 © BSIP Agency/Index Stock; p. 31 © CMSP; p. 33 © Barry Sweet/Associated Press; p. 33 © Hulton-Deutsch Collection/Corbis; p. 37 © CMSP; p. 40 © A. Pasieka/Photo Researchers, Inc.

Series Design

Laura Murawski

Layout

Danielle Goldblatt